I0412510

A Young Gentleman's Guide To Losing Your Virginity

Everything You Haven't Been Told And Need To Know

by C.W. Pollard

A Gentleman's Sexual Compendium Series
Publication

Copyright Notice

Copyright © Overunity Publications 2011. All rights reserved. None of the materials in this publication may be used, reproduced or transmitted, in whole or in part, in any form or by any means, electronic or mechanical, including photocopying, recording or the use of any information storage and retrieval system, without permission in writing from the publisher. To request such permission and for further inquiries, contact Overunity Publications at contact@overunitypublications.com

First Edition: 2011

ISBN 978-1468019179

Trademark Disclaimer

Product names, logos, brands, URLs, web site links, and other trademarks featured or referred to within this publication or within any supplemental or related materials are the property of their respective trademark holders. These trademark holders are not affiliated with the author or publisher and the trademark holders do not sponsor or endorse our materials.

Copyright Acknowledgment

Photographs attributed to a third party are the property of such third party and are used here by permission. All such attributed photographs are subject to the copyright claims of each respective owner.

Legal Disclaimer

Although the author and the publisher believe that the included information is accurate and useful, nothing contained in this publication can be considered professional advice on any legal or accounting matter. You must consult a licensed attorney or accountant if you want professional advice that is appropriate to your particular situation.

Losing your virginity is a complicated process that is a combination of wild luck, plucky exuberance and all the mistruths you have picked up along your quest to get the pussy. When I finally was poised to lose my cherry my head was swimming with information my friends had told me (mostly lies), my parent's sex books from the 70s had told me (mostly weird), and what public sex education had told me (mostly useless). It was a comedy of errors, high hopes and it was over much, much sooner than I had expected or she would have liked.

Let's face it. Losing your virginity is one of those subjects that's hard to deal with. You don't want to hear about your dad's first time. Most of your friends are lying and have no idea what they are talking about anyway. Plus, you sure as hell don't need to know what a fallopian tube is to get your rocks off. So what does a plucky young lad do? Well, you buy this book. In it you will find the practical, no nonsense information you need to get it wet for the first time. Plus, you don't have to cringe or be embarrassed. You can read this on your time and learn exactly what to expect, what to do and what not to do. This is the book you have been looking for since you first knew what a pussy was and what you wanted to do with it.

Before Losing Your Virginity

Chance Favors The Prepared

So you have decided that it is time to lose your virginity. You, as are ready to embrace the world and to seize your sexual destiny. It's time. You may even have a woman who is willing to let you fuck her. What more is there to do? Well, trust me. There is a fair amount of planning that you need to do. In this enterprise, chance favors the prepared and it is the prepared man that loses his virginity. So before you go out and try to lose that virginity, let's go over a few steps you need to check off first.

Admit How You Are Feeling To Yourself

Sun Tsu, the famous Chinese philosopher said that "Battles are won or lost in the temples, before they are ever fought in the field.". What does this mean and what bearing could it possibly have on the subject of losing your virginity? Well, what this means is that, if you are a general, you want your troops heads to be in the right place before they go into battle. You too, want your head to be in the right place before you try and lose your virginity.

Let's face it, losing your virginity is a big, often scary deal. It is very emotional. You are crossing one of the last hurdles to manhood. It can also be scary. I was terrified about a woman seeing me naked for the first time, or that it would go wrong. There is nothing wrong with admitting, to yourself and only yourself, that you are a little scared too.

Take some time out of your life and ponder on this subject. When I am faced with a difficult challenge, I like to identify where and what potential problems exist. That allows me to calmly, and rationally plan how I will overcome each of them in turn. I did it when I taught myself to drive a manual transmission. I do it when I have had job interviews. I sure as hell did it when losing my virginity was imminent. Doing this doesn't make the fear go away, but it definitely lets you manage it and it tends to take the power of the fears away.

As a bottom line, it is OK if your are nervous. I would be shocked if you weren't. However, you will be OK. Identity why you are nervous and figure out how you will deal with the fears that you have. Win this battle now, in the temple (you mind), before you fight in the field (have sex in the bedroom).

A Practical Lesson In Anatomy

You need to be familiar with female anatomy before you try and lose your virginity. This is an absolutely critical part of your training and you need to spend some time getting to know what everything is and where you can find it. Most importantly, you need to know that a woman's pussy encompasses everything in the diagram above and all of it is sensitive. You can give her pleasure many different ways through her many different parts and a good lover will know how.

Before we dive in, I want to make sure that you are aware of a simple fact of developmental biology. This is the fact that all humans, men and women, start out physically female. It is a hormone reaction that causes an embryo to develop into a male. Mother Nature is practical and all she does is modify existing female anatomy to make a male. Of course, I am massively oversimplifying this, but you get the point. So, for example, the clitoris elongates and becomes a penis, vaginal lips come together and fuse to become a scrotum (that's where that seam comes from), etc., etc,.

This means that when you think of a woman's anatomy, you really can think of it in terms of your own junk. For example, to understand how to touch and please her clitoris, think about how it feels when the tip of your penis is touched. The same delicate touch that feels good on the head of your penis also feels good to her clit.

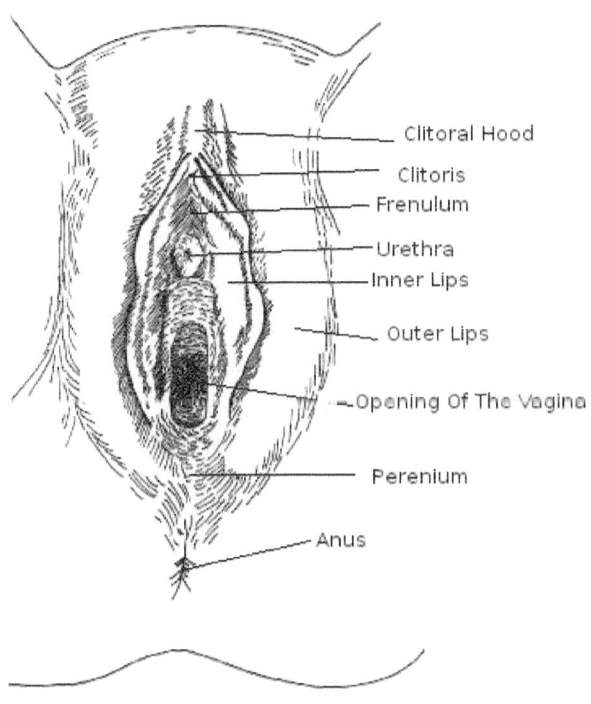

Clitoral Hood

Clitoris

Frenulum

Urethra

Inner Lips

Outer Lips

Opening Of The Vagina

Perenium

Anus

Now that we are all well schooled in developmental biology, let's get started in this crash course of woman's anatomy.

Start at the top of the diagram and we will work our way down. At the very top of her vagina, you will find her clitoris. This is the most famous tourist destination in a woman's pussy, and you should pay a lot of attention to this little organ. Now, remember, that a man's penis is simply a modified clitoris, or conversely, a clitoris is just a tiny penis. They are built along very similar lines. There is a tremendous amount of nerve endings in both. They are, however, much more concentrated in the clitoris. Stimulation of these nerves in both sexes are what gives everyone an orgasm. In men it results in ejaculation, in women, contractions of her vaginal muscles. In both sexes it feels great. The clitoris even swells when a woman is sexually excited just like the penis in men.

Now most men think the clitoris is really just a tiny button that they need to push. This is absolutely wrong. The clitoris is actually extends back and up on the woman's pussy and is protected by a layer of skin that can be pulled back. This skin is often called the clitoral hood and serves the same purpose as a foreskin on men, in that it protects the sensitive tissue. By placing your hand just above the woman's pussy (she is lying on her back with her legs spread) and gently pulling upward you can actually expose more of the clitoris. This exposes more nerve endings to your sucking, licking and fingering. Some women enjoy this and others will find it too intense.

Below the clitoris and inside the vaginal lips, above the urethra, you will find the vaginal frenulum. This is a soft, tender patch of skin that most people don't pay any attention to. This is a great area to stroke (after you have wet your finger with saliva). This is a stimulating act that will not lead to orgasm, however, it will very much heighten her arousal. That is a great secret right there.

The vaginal lips are another set of major features in the pussy that you need to be familiar with. There are two sets. The first is the labia majora. These are the lips that are often called camel toes. They are well developed and often covered with hair. The purpose of these lips are to protect all the delicate and tender bits immediately surrounding the vagina. It is by no means uncommon for you to need to spread these lips slightly with your fingers or tongue to gain access to the pussy itself.

However, these are great for foreplay. One of my favorite subtly arousing techniques to to stroke the labia majora with my index and ring finger up and down. Do this very slightly so that your fingers are almost just tickling this area. As a more advanced technique, you can also **GENTLY** pinch the whole vaginal area between your thumb and the first knuckle of your index finger.

Once you have done this, you can slowly move her whole pussy up (towards her clitoris) and down (towards her anus). This feels great over the whole pussy, and again, heightens the sense of arousal. Start your movements small and keep eye contact with her while you are doing this. This will increase your emotional connection and at the same time tune you into how she is enjoying the stimulation.

Inside the outer lips of the pussy (labia majora) you will find another set of lips. These are the labia minora or inner lips. These folds of tissue are immediately on the sides of the vaginal opening itself. These are very sensitive but they are also delicate. She will respond well to stimulation in this area, however, just like the clitoris, start softly and work up the pressure while you pay attention to her body movements. You don't want to hurt anything. The inner lips are also your guide to the clitoris itself. The clitoris is usually (not all women have the same pussy) located just below where the inner lips join at the top of the pussy. You can almost always follow them with your tongue or finger and they will lead you where you want to go.

The vaginal opening is contained inside her inner lips. This is where your penis goes during intercourse (I'm really hoping you already knew that). However, it can play a huge role in foreplay as well. However, you should really not spend a lot of time here with your mouth. There are nerve endings in the vagina for sure, however, you are really best inserting your fingers or a dildo in this area. (We'll talk more about this later.) Women love to have the feeling of being filled and simply inserting a finger or two will greatly enhance the oral sex. However, your mouth should spend most of its time either teasing the lips or stimulating her clitoris.

Below her vagina you will find her perenium. This is simple a patch of skin that divides her pussy from her anus. This is definitely a fun area to tease her with. You can put kisses here all day, however, there are no large amounts of nerve ends in this area.

Below her perenium is her anus. We will talk more about the anus later too.

Planning For Foreplay

Another failure of sex education is often (almost 100% of the time) the failure to teach and communicate the importance of foreplay. Take it from me, this is important so pay attention. Foreplay is everything that leads up to actual penetration. Women so often joke about how poor their lovers perform in the foreplay department, but it is usually just their way of saying that they don't get enough. You, as a refined young gentleman eager to set out on his maiden sexual voyage, however, are going to do your part to reverse that trend by paying attention to what I am about to tell you.

Foreplay is important for two simple reasons. First, it turns both men and women on physically and gets our cocks and pussies ready for the physical act of love. Secondly, as the majority of sexual arousal takes place in the brain, it allows our minds to get good and turned on too.

As a man, you are aware of the physical effects of arousal. When your girlfriend has teasingly kissed your neck and maybe chest in the past, your cock gets hard. You may have also noticed that little drip of precum that always forms on the tip of your cock too. That is the sign that you are all set to go, physically speaking. At that point, your penis is secreting your contribution to the lubricants that are necessary for comfortable sexual intercourse.

Now, your lubrication contribution, as a man is going to be pitifully small in the grand scheme of things. This is the important part so pay attention here. <u>The majority of the lubricant that is needed for comfortable sex to occur is going to come from her. Pussies are self lubricating. Foreplay is what you do and the amount of time you spend getting her excited so her pussy will get nice and slippery for your cock.</u> Why is this important to you? Well, because if you don't spend enough time on foreplay her pussy will dry, it will hurt in a very short amount of time, and she won't fuck you anymore because you make her pussy hurt. A gentleman always makes sure to spend a lot of time on foreplay for the comfort of his partner so she will fuck him more in the future. Got it? OK. Good. <u>Make sure her pussy is good and wet before you stick it in by engaging in lots of foreplay.</u>

Now you're probably scratching your head wondering just what you are supposed to do and for how long you are supposed to do it. Don't panic! I am going to tell you what you need to know there too.

The first and most important part of foreplay is kissing. You should kiss your lover a lot and all over her body. There is something magic in the kiss that we still don't understand. Seriously, science can't explain why we like it, yet we all do. So, go with it and enjoy. Kiss her on the lips and make out with her in a way that would be just obnoxious in public. Savor every minute of it and lose yourself in that magic.

When you find yourself naked with you luscious femme fatale and the time for losing your cherry fast approaches, also make an effort to kiss all over her body. Take your time, kiss her lips a lot in between, but then get back to exploring all of her curves with your tongue and lips. Yes, I mean all of her curves, peaks and valleys. No woman that I have ever met will have any problem with her lover giving her this kind of attention and she will frequently melt. Just remember, every kiss makes that pussy of hers just a little wetter and slipperier for you and that means better sex, longer sex and sex more often.

At this point, a lot of young men make the decision to go for the gold and try to eat their lover's pussy. This is great. They want to make their lover happy by trying to please her. This is fine, great actually, but you need to go into this act of foreplay with no goals. Chances are very slim that you will be able to make her cum. You can try, and if you want to, I recommend reading my other book "The Secret Art Of Eating Pussy: Tips & Tricks To Please Her Every Time" before you make the attempt. Now, I said chances are slim that you will make her cum, but she will really appreciate the effort and thought and it will definitely make her wetter. Just remember – no goals and no expectations.

Fingering is another great act of foreplay. You should finger any woman you are trying to make love to a lot as well. Fingering, again, is not something that is ever really taught to you. I am going to take a few lines here and try to give you a basic course in fingering that will put you light years ahead of many of your peers.

First and foremost with fingering, forget the concept of "finger bang". This is a very common mistake. Many young men seem to think that for a woman to enjoy fingering, you need to, essentially, fuck her with your finger. Nope. Dead wrong. This can actually be uncomfortable in the wrong hands (a bit of a pun intended there). Instead, we are going to focus on rubbing and gentle penetration only.

Now, before you employ either of the fingering techniques that i am going to instruct you on, I want to make sure that you know to wet your finger. Yes, you need to lick any finger to get it wet before you go and touch any of her sensitive pussy bits. If yo don't, the dry skin of your finger can stick to the wet tissues of her pussy and cause a bit of discomfort. So, as a gentleman, we always make sure to get a good amount of saliva on our fingers. Saliva, for reference, is the best natural sexual lubricant. You can do this discreetly if you want, but I find that the act of consideration is greatly appreciated when our lovers see it. Plus, seeing you lick your finger before sticking it in her pussy is arousing too.

Now, the first fingering technique that I am going to instruct you on is external fingering. External fingering is rubbing the external parts of her pussy with your fingers. You should use the index, middle and ring fingers of your dominant hand. (NOTE: You should be kissing her the whole time you are doing this.) Take and lick the palm side of these three fingers to apply a generous amount of saliva on them. Then reach between your lover's legs and apply the palm side of these three fingers to her pussy. In a quirk of human anatomy, these three fingers should just about cover her whole pussy. Now, apply **gentle** pressure over the whole area of her pussy. Start light, as you can always increase pressure based on her reactions.

Think of this as the equivalent of her putting her hand around your cock. She doesn't even have to move it for it to turn you on does she? In fact, that act often makes you incredibly horny and you might even feel a bit teased. Well, now the shoe is on the other foot so to speak. Just putting your hand there will feel good and excite her. Your paying attention to her and her puss. This, in turn makes her pussy more lubricated and closer to being ready for sex.

Now, with the palm side of your index, middle and ring fingers flush against her pussy, and a little light pressure being applied, move your fingers in a circular motion. Clockwise or counterclockwise is fine. There is no secret move. Again, start slow. You can always speed up, again, based on how she reacts.

You might be tempted to go digging and find her clitoris and work her to a couple of orgasms. DON'T! Instead, apply the pressure to her outer vaginal lips and just move her whole pussy in a circular motion. This is like here gently, slowly stroking your cock. Trust me, she will be very turned on by this subtle, yet very effective manual stimulation technique.

Now, we can move on to internal fingering. Of course, during all of this manual stimulation you should be kissing your lover. This dramatically heightens the excitement and makes her feel close to you. This is what you want. Also, if you are feeling drawn to and closer to her at the same time - great.

Internal fingering is when you insert your fingers into the vagina itself. Again, we are not looking for the clitoris here, or trying to make her cum, or to "fingerbang" her. We are simply trying to provide stimulation to her pussy in order to excite her and cause her vagina to lubricate.

Internal fingering always begins with external fingering. You should always be in the process of externally fingering her before you move on to internal fingering. It is a very natural progression. Also, before moving to internal fingering, you should always bring your hand back up for more saliva. Yes, it all sounds technical and a little messy, but sex is often wet and messy. This time, put your index finger and your middle finger all the way in your mouth, you need to get the whole of both finger good and wet.

Resume external fingering for a moment or two, however, this time, move your index and middle finger towards the middle of her vagina. You are looking for her vaginal opening. I am going to assume this is your first time looking for this, so bear with me if I seem a tad patronizing. The vaginal opening is located at the bottom of her pussy (like we talked about) just above where the vaginal lips come together. It gets really wet there, so if in your probing you feel it getting drier, you are on the wrong path. Go back. Look for it with the tip of your index finger. When you think you've found it, probe it a little up to the first knuckle. If it goes in all the way, you're there. Once you've found it, trust me, you won't have trouble after that.

Now, slowly and gently, slip in the whole of your index finger. When fingering, the palm side of your hand should always be pointing up towards her clitoris, not her ass. Now, this is where some good technique really pays off. Here, with your index finger all the way inside your lover's pussy you might be tempted to just start jamming it in and out. Don't. Instead, like before, just apply subtle pressure into her vagina (don't worry your hand won't slip up there). Start slow and easy and apply more based on her reactions. You can also move your finger around in little circular motions. Imagine trying to draw a circle with the tip of your finger that is the size of a nickel. That's perfect. As she becomes comfortable with one finger, you can feel free to slip in your index finger. Don't change how you are moving them. Apply the same gentle pressure and draw the same sized circle with the tips of both fingers. Just don't fingerbang!

Now, with all of this kissing and all of this fingering, you should have gotten her very turned on by now. Conveniently enough, with your fingers in her pussy, you are also in a great position to determine if her pussy is wet enough. If your fingers are moving in and out smoothly with little to no friction, congratulate yourself, you have made a woman very wet and ready for sex!

Now, just because she is ready for sex, doesn't mean that you have to go and slip it in. Instead, leap ahead a few years in maturity and sexual technique and wait for her to tell you to slip it in. Young women are very used to having a guy just slip it in and cum in two seconds. No concern being given to their pleasure at all. Instead, set yourself apart and wait. Enjoy the moment and the magic of your first time. When she tells you she's ready, that is your moment. Then, by all means, slip it in and accept your destiny and manhood. Trust me, when she goes and tells all her friends about how you waited until she was ready and how good you are at foreplay, those young women will look at you in a whole new, very curious, light. You might have a few more chances to practice your foreplay skills before things are all over.

You Nails

It so rarely occurs to a young man who is trying to lose his cherry, but your nails are very important to sex. Actually, to be more accurate, they can be problematic to sex if you don't take care of them. Here is the problem. Long nails and nails with sharp corners can be very rough on a woman's delicate areas. You can scrape, scratch and slice if you are not careful and this hurts a lot!

What you need to do is go to the health and beauty section of your favorite retailer and buy some emery boards. Those are those little sandpaper boards that women use when they get a manicure. Guess what! You, as a horny young gentleman virgin, in the hopes of losing your cherry, are going to use them too. Go buy a ten pack, they're very cheap. Open them. Use them. Use them a lot. Make sure your nails are both short and well rounded. Keep them that way all the time. When the time comes and you are ready, you'll thank me.

Maintain Your Space

I lost my virginity a long time ago and most of my friends did too. Not long ago, a few months in fact, I was out at a club with some of my friends. One of my wingmen was been fortunate enough to meet and eager, young woman who wanted to go back to his place for some adult recreation. He was amped. He was horny. He was eager. However, he is also a little dumb. He had not counted on this possibility occurring and he had left his bedroom a disaster. I'm talking skid marked undies and used jack off magazines lying all over the place. Exactly the kind of setup that is all but guaranteed to kill any woman's girly boner.

I'm telling you this story because it illustrates a valuable lesson that many men my own age have still not learned. If you want to get laid, even if it's only your first time, you need to keep your space (i.e. Your bedroom) nice and tidy. It should be presentable. Women are like cats, they don't like messes. They usually won't fuck you if your bedroom is messy. So, when you have decided to lose your virginity, you also need to make it a habit to keep your room, if not your apartment, nice and clean and always ready to bring a woman back to. Learn that lesson now and you will be well ahead of many of the men my age, let alone yours.

No Spicy Food Beforehand

I would have lost my virginity a few days sooner than I did if it wasn't for that damn taco. See, what happened was this. I wanted to have a nice dinner with my special lady friend, before we went back to my empty parent's house for sweet love making. I was a line cook at the time and I was spending a lot of my weekly paycheck in this sumptuous feast. Well, I was young and dumb and I didn't know any better. I loaded up my already spicy taco with the finest Mexican hot sauces I could. I ate. I savored. I enjoyed.

Then, I went down (poorly) on my special lady friend. Bad idea. That pesky capsicum (what makes peppers spicy) must still have been in my mouth a bit. What I did without knowing it was lick it all over my girlfriend's pussy. It burned. She had to go and wash he hoo hah off and I'll tell you, when she got back she was in no mood for first time loving. Cock blocked again.

So, free advice here, when you are wining and dining your lady before your first time, think bland food.

Foot Rubs Are A Key That Opens Many Doors

I don't have a son. I don't know that I ever will. I also don't have a little brother. However, if I had either of these family relations and they came to their trusty dad or older brother and said "How do I get laid?"; I would look them in the eye and say "foot rubs".

I'm serious. The foot rub has to be one of the fastest, easiest, and most underused of all seduction techniques. I have made it a little bit of a life goal to get the word out. It won't hurt anyone. The ladies get more foot rubs and the guys get more ladies. Everyone is a winner.

My scientific research as to why this happens is still inconclusive, but I think it goes something like this. Women's feet are errogenous zones. That is to say that they get turned on when someone touches their feet. Their feet get as sore as ours do, so they want foot rubs. When a man rubs their feet he is easing their pain, showing he cares and physically arousing her all at the same time. This combination creates a situation that is just perfect to turn into lovemaking. All it needs is a spark.

So go on and offer to rub your girlfriend's feet. Just ask. If you need lotion, I'm sure she'll have some. Women always have lotion. Don't try and turn it into sex, just make it about rubbing her feet and making her feel good. Forget about sex all together. This will make the chances of sex all the more likely. I know it's weird but go with it. If it doesn't work the firs time just keep trying. Trust me, in the end it will work. It always does.

Wear A Condom No Matter What

I'm going to keep this section really brief. There are a lot of bugs out there and unfortunately, a young man can't be too careful. Even if your girlfriend is a virgin like you, there is always lurking pregnancy – the easiest STD to catch. So keep it simple wear a condom all the time no matter what. Don't try pulling out at the last minute. Don't rely on her not being fertile at this time of the month. Don't run out of condoms and roll the dice. Wear a condom 100% of the time! OK. I'm done with that.

Keep Your Sex Locker Full

Another failing that sex education commits is that you are often not taught on condoms, sex toys and lubes. You should make sure, that at the very least, you have plenty of condoms available to you when you plan to lose your virginity. I'm talking 50+ or so. You laugh, and think that one is all you need. Well, I laugh at the man who runs out of condoms and has to try and find a store in a deserted seaside town that sells condoms at 11:30 at night and can't find one. Alright, I'll confess. I was that man and it sucked. I was nineteen and stupid and stuck with a case of blueballs that wouldn't quit that night. Don't make the same mistake.

You also need to make sure that you have a variety of condoms available. At the very least go for unlubricated, lubricated and spermicidally lubricated. When I first lost my virginity I was wearing a lubricated condom. Lubricated condoms add just a little bit of slipperiness in case she is nervous and dry or you ignore my instructions on foreplay (those will come shortly). Call 'em cheater condoms. Well, in my case it was too damn slippery down there (I was as big a proponent of foreplay then as I am now). I'm mean an oil slick on an icy road. Well, I was forced to switch to the unlibricated before I could get traction and break the plane and claim the touchdown. Spermicidally lubricated are great for added birth control, however, the lube tastes awful. If you plan to try and go down on her afterwards, I would stick with the unlubricated or just plain unlubricated. Either way, you should have a lot of all three types.

You should also have some lubrication on hand, in a bottle. There are plenty of commercially available lubricants. You can find these, along with all the condoms you will ever need at your local pharmacy/grocery store. You don't have to go to your local dildo store to find the basic necessities of losing your virginity.

One last note on lubes. Make sure that it is a water based lubricant. Oil based lubricants, like petroleum jelly or baby oil, are corrosive to condoms. This means that the condoms won't protect your from herpes or babies. Also, the lubes can be irritating to sensitive tissues. Any water based lubricant will advertise that it is just that on the bottle. Just take the time to look for it.

Arranging Alone Time

The most critical challenge that you are likely to face as a man looking to lose his virginity is to arrange some alone time with you and your chosen lady. This can be tricky. Parents show up at the wrong time. Roommates plans can get scratched and husbands can come home early. All of this can ruin your first time. They might catch you balls deep and you have to run out the window (happened to a friend of mine...or so he claimed) or worse yet they can come home just as you are ready to slip it in and totally cockblock you. One of your last milestones before becoming a man will be to figure out a way for the two of you to get one on one.

I can't tell you exactly how to do this. However, man has evolved a very large brain (in my opinion just to figure out more ways to get laid) and it is up to you to use it. Your situation is unique, but I will offer a few suggestions for making one on one time a reality. With a little luck, these will inspire you to your own unique solution and you'll be balls deep in no time.

The most obvious solution is a hotel. These can be a little pricey if your girl insists on romance. A nice downtown hotel can cost several hundred dollars for the night. However, the romance can often make the difference between getting another handy and finally losing your virginity. So spend the extra money for the romance if you go the hotel route. Even better, if you can arrange the transportation and swing the hotel bill, is a getaway in your area. I'm sure there's something in your area. Think waterfall, lake, beach or mountain. Any one of these will do and can possibly tip the balance with a little romantic slight of hand.

One last note on lubes. Make sure that it is a water based lubricant. Oil based lubricants, like petroleum jelly or baby oil, are corrosive to condoms. This means that the condoms won't protect your from herpes or babies. Also, the lubes can be irritating to sensitive tissues. Any water based lubricant will advertise that it is just that on the bottle. Just take the time to look for it.

Arranging Alone Time

The most critical challenge that you are likely to face as a man looking to lose his virginity is to arrange some alone time with you and your chosen lady. This can be tricky. Parents show up at the wrong time. Roommates plans can get scratched and husbands can come home early. All of this can ruin your first time. They might catch you balls deep and you have to run out the window (happened to a friend of mine...or so he claimed) or worse yet they can come home just as you are ready to slip it in and totally cockblock you. One of your last milestones before becoming a man will be to figure out a way for the two of you to get one on one.

I can't tell you exactly how to do this. However, man has evolved a very large brain (in my opinion just to figure out more ways to get laid) and it is up to you to use it. Your situation is unique, but I will offer a few suggestions for making one on one time a reality. With a little luck, these will inspire you to your own unique solution and you'll be balls deep in no time.

The most obvious solution is a hotel. These can be a little pricey if your girl insists on romance. A nice downtown hotel can cost several hundred dollars for the night. However, the romance can often make the difference between getting another handy and finally losing your virginity. So spend the extra money for the romance if you go the hotel route. Even better, if you can arrange the transportation and swing the hotel bill, is a getaway in your area. I'm sure there's something in your area. Think waterfall, lake, beach or mountain. Any one of these will do and can possibly tip the balance with a little romantic slight of hand.

Now, hotels can be expensive and I know that when I lost my cherry, I could barely scrape two nickels together. A cheaper option is always camping. I didn't lose my virginity camping, but several of the sexual milestones on that road were achieved on a beach campout. This also has the benefit of having romance about it since most camping is again, lake adjacent or at the beach etc. - plus it's cheap if not free. Girls love campfires too!

Patience can often provide what you need and cannot obtain. You can wait until you parents or roommates go out of town and try for some alone time then. The holidays can be a perfect time for that. Wait for your parents to go to grandmas, tell them your boss is a dick and making you work and then hang out at the house together. Maybe they are going on vacation. Well, in that case, stay home. Tell them you don't care about Aruba. Trust me, sex is better anyway.

Find a first time sex partner who lives alone or whose housemates leave on a frequent basis, or perhaps a husband who travels and then pounce. We will talk about how to find these secret MILFs, cougars and big girls in just a bit.

As a last resort, forget the need for a bed just look for privacy. I mean anywhere. This can be in the stockroom late at night when you are doing inventory. This can be in the church rec room during services or in the gym late at night. Whatever it it just needs to be private. A car can work, but anyone who has ever really fucked in a sedan will tell you it is never comfortable. If you do plan on using the car, think van or station wagon with sleeping bags. That part about sleeping bags is important. Cars get cold. In the end a car isn't a pretty win but it will do if that's all the privacy you can find. The only other problem is that it is unromantic and you may have a bit more selling to do it with your girl. But it is possible.

As a last resort, try a mid-afternoon getaway picnic on a sunny day. Go to a park that doesn't seem busy, find a discrete spot and see what happens. Try making out and see where it leads. If you feel the mood is right and the coast is clear, well try your luck. You'll be brief anyway. This act, is actually a bit naughty and you will be surprised how easy it can be to sell a woman on a sex act, especially when its a little risque. She may chomp at the bit for you to bend her over behind a tree. Just for convenience, have her wear a skirt and make the panties optional.

Hopefully these few notes will give you a few ideas and insights that will allow you to craft a solution to your alone time problem. Nothing less than your sex life hangs in the balance so I'm sure you're inspired already.

A Gentleman Let's It Happen. He Doesn't Pressure

I have and have had a lot of girlfriends, both romantically and platonically. We have had many personal conversations and one way or another the subject of our first times comes up eventually. It's always been a mixed bag subject but I have noticed a persistent theme. In this case, the theme is that many of these women have regretted their first time partners and only lost their virginities under a great deal of pressure. I won't say that I was completely immune to putting of this pressure either. I am no innocent. However, if I were writing this document to myself, as a virgin many years ago, I would advise myself to leave the pressure behind and let it happen when it happens. Patience is hard when you have a hardon ten or fifteen times a day, but in the end it may be worth it. So seduce your partner, don't pressure her. That's my advice on that subject. Take it or leave it

Understanding Her Point Of View Is Key

Losing your virginity is a hugely important moment to you. However, I find that I would be remiss in my responsibilities if I did not pause for a moment and try to offer you a little perspective on women, and their take on sex and virginity. First of all, let me make it very obvious and clear that women enjoy sex just as much as men do and are just as curious.

The first point that you may not have considered where virginity is concerned is pain. If you are losing your virginity all you are thinking about is slipping your throbbing member into the warm, wet, inviting pussy of a woman of your acquaintance. She, on the other hand, when thinking about losing her virginity, is thinking about how much it will hurt. She knows from friends, parents, and school that it will hurt a bit. Just how much, she's not sure. That uncertainty can definitely create a bit of anxiety on her part. Try and see it from her point of view. Imagine it's your first night in prison and you know someone is going to rape you in the ass. Forget all the psychological damage, and just think about how you would feel. It's nice and tight and innocent back there. You know that your cellmate is going to hurt it, but you just aren't sure how much. How eager would you be? I'm willing to bet that you would be a little reluctant too.

Next, she is worried about pregnancy. Women are the ones who have to bear the physical side effects of sex. She's scared she'll ruin her life with a pregnancy. Her mind has been filled with after school specials and horror stories from her parents and friends about women who "gave it up" and then got "knocked up". She also would be the one who would need to make a decision about keeping the baby or getting an abortion. Yes, you could be a stand up guy and be there with her, but in the end, the final decision is hers and that is scary as hell. No woman ever wants to have to make that choice.

Lastly, she's afraid of being a slut, even to you. Yes, you read that last part right. Women are under tremendous social pressure to act appropriately. This means that they often have to keep their sexuality under raps. She is thinking that if she gives up the pussy to easily, you will think she's a slut and will then not want anything to do with her after you've fucked her. Truth be told, for many young men, she's right. Her reputation is very important and she wants to protect it at all cost.

She is also doing some counting. Women look at their sexual history very differently than men. Men look at the number of sexual partners as something to brag about and the more he wants to tell people about it. The more pussies a cock has been in, the more virile the man, the more desirable he is as a lover. Women look at their count like a car. You can only get so many miles out of a car's engine. Well, she can only put so many cocks into her pussy before it's all used up (in her mind). Women actually lower and lie about the number of lovers they've had to get around this. Like rolling back the odometer on a car. So, to make the decision to sleep with you, she has to add some miles to her engine and that of course lowers its value. Now, of course by value, I mean her self worth and they way society and future lovers and husbands see her. This is all very much in her mind too before she ever decides to sleep with you.

Now, all of this is not to say that women don't want to climb on top of you and fuck your brains out. Trust me, they do, like I said. These last few paragraphs have hopefully just made you a little more aware of the fairer sex and will hopefully make you a better, more empathetic lover in the process.

Thoughts On Cougar Hunting & Chub Chasing

Now, I am just putting this out there for you to consider. Part of what I am doing here is offering you ideas that you may not have thought of yet in your quest to lose your virginity. So keep that in mind. However, if you are having trouble seducing and making sweet love to the women in your age or peer group, you may need to look for some other, different yet equally enjoyable fruit. By this of course I mean older women and fat girls. There I said it.

Most people that read that first paragraph would take something negative away from it. On the contrary! I have been the lover of both older women and fat women (sometimes the same woman) and I will tell you that I respected and enjoyed my time with all of them. The reason that I mention it is that they are, statistically speaking, simply much easier to have sex with. I'm not a psychologist so I won't even try to explain, but from my own empirical evidence, it's true. Maybe part of it is that they are grateful for the attention of a younger man and are unaccustomed to receiving it.

When I was a much younger man (well under 20) I met a woman who was 42. She was married and unhappy. Now, I am no proponent of infidelity, but at the time I hadn't gotten my dick wet and didn't know any better. Well we were hot and heavy for some time. Every day after school, I would rush home to have a dirty phone conversation with her (alas we didn't have all the fun technology that you do now). Your imagination can fill in the datails, but I will say, that i had a lot of fun with that 42 year old woman.

Another time, through the miracle of a young internet I made the acquaintance of a divorcee with two kids. She was younger, I want to say about 35 at the time, but she was a big gal. I would say 280 if she was a pound. Now, I can assure you that though she was a big woman, the two of us got along swimmingly and had a lot of fun when her kids were at their dad's. Really, all she wanted was an adult playmate which was perfect for me. No strings, just dirty fun. I think she was enjoying the freedom of her new divorce. I smile now, as I write and think about her.

My point here is that if you keep an open mind in terms of looking for a woman to lose your cherry to, your quest can be a lot easier. All too often we focus on the ideal and overlook the possible and easily obtainable. Keep an open mind in your search for your first and you may be surprised what fate throws in your path. I was and still am to this day.

With the march of technology, one of the best places to meet older and bigger gals eager to meet you, is still the internet. I am not going to list any websites, I am sure you know where to look and what to do. I will just recommend that you spend a night or two exploring these options. Keep an open mind and fate may lead you through a door you never expected and will never forget.

I will say, just so there is no confusion about my intention or my glib section heading; no matter what treat your partner with dignity and respect like a lady deserves. Never forget a gentleman treats the ladies right.

Speaking Of Prostitutes...

I want to address a subject that comes up fairly often with horny young men. That is the subject of prostitutes. Every know and again, a young man gets the idea that it would be a lot easier to lose his cherry to a prostitute rather than the girl next door. On the surface, there is some logic to this. A prostitute is a done deal and there is no romancing. Plus, there's much less awkwardness. You'll never have to see her again. Maybe you'll get the chance on that family cruise to Mexico or that vacation to the Netherlands this summer.

However, when you get down to the basics, there are four solid reasons that you should not go to a prostitute to lose your virginity (or really ever).

One, prostitution is usually illegal. Now, I am not morally opposed to prostitution on it's face. I am a libertarian and I think that a consenting adult woman should be able to make the adult decision to engage in sex for money. That being said, the law in many countries prohibits prostitution and you don't want to wind up in any legal trouble. That would just mean you have a fine, community service and still have a raging chub to boot.

Secondly, prostitution is often unsafe. There are two prongs to this argument. First, you never know where a prostitute has been. Maybe she is some washed up lot lizard who has been blowing truckers for meth until just before you met her. You don't know anything about her history or how long it has been since her herpes broke out. I'm being glib, but STDs are real and you can wind up with them, for life, from hookers. There is still no cure for HIV.

Also, because prostitution is illegal, the people who engage in it are criminals. This makes them much more willing to use violence at times. Consult your local law enforcement and I am sure that they will be perfectly happy to provide you with many examples of hookers robbing their johns either by trickery or force. Extortion comes up too and there are many scams that I won't even mention. Long story short, when you mix it up with prostitutes, you tend to put yourself in a bad position. Just don't.

Now, while I mentioned that in principle I have not objection to prostitution, the reality is that prostitution is very often, immoral. Prostitution, in the real world, all too often involves exploitation. All too often women are forced into the trade. Often, prostitution is nothing more than sexual slavery. Frequently, the women in prostitution rings are also underage and strung out on drugs. This is not something that any young gentleman should be a party too.

Lastly, as cliche as it sounds, your first time should be special. There is a lot of emotion and magic tied up in the experience of losing your virginity. Good or bad, you will never forget it. It is something that you will also feel much better about if you work to achieve it. I laugh now when I think of the comedy of errors that led up to my first time and how fast it was all over. However, I can still remember it clearly and fondly. I wouldn't trade that awkward experience (remember, I didn't have this book) for anything. If you go to a prostitute it is a lot like cheating.

Any woman's studies major who reads this will cringe, but I think a man (and that's how I'm going to treat you) will get this analogy. It's a lot like fishing. Yes, you can go to the store and buy a fish. You will have the same fish as if you had gotten up early and caught it, but the magic won't be there. In losing your virginity, just like fishing, the true magic and what makes it special, is in the getting, not in the having. Remember that!

While You're Using Your Virginity

Hold On. This Will Only Take A Second

Before I lost my virginity, I was a prodigious masturbator. I was young and chocked full of hormones and sexual enthusiasm. (Just so we're clear here, I still am and do not pretend to be otherwise). I would rub it out many times a day. My junk was well conditioned and I felt that I had decent control. I was relatively certain that when the time came to actually slip my wedding tackle into a willing woman came along, I would be able to last a respectful amount of time. How wrong I was.

Honestly, you need to come to accept the fact that your first time will be over before you know it. This happens, simply because you are so excited at the prospect of actually having sex with a woman, that your body just gets overwhelmed. You are going to slip it in, pump it a few times and before you know it you're cumming. Maybe humans even evolved that way. Mother Nature figured that if you ever got a chance to fuck a woman you should cum quick before the two of you got interrupted. That way, statistically, there is the highest chance of reproduction. Practical from Mother Nature's standpoint, but a bit of a pain in the ass for any young man.

A lot of men, including me are afraid of this. They (still including me) are afraid that their partner will think them less of a man, or may even laugh at them. Maybe their girlfriend will think that they are a poor lover because they are also a "two pump chump".

Well, since you are going to be a two pump chump your first time (nothing we can do to fix that) you need to accept this and spin it. What I mean, is that we need to turn this potential blow to our ego into a compliment to our partner's. This in turn will defuse the situation and any embarrassment associated with it. What does all this mean?

Well, it means this. Imagine you have just lost your virginity and you have just cum in three seconds flat. You look at your girlfriend and in her mind she is debating whether this is good or bad. What you do is you look her in the eye and you say something like "Oh man, I'm sorry that was so quick but you just turned me on so much! You're so beautiful.". Then you kiss her.

What this does is it turns your quick draw act into a compliment to her ego. Women love compliments and she wants to believe it. So her mind will just turn the fact that you came in three seconds flat into a compliment and everything is fine. You were simply overwhelmed by her beauty and sex appeal. Case closed. Get your cuddle on and feel good. You just lost your cherry and complimented your lover at the same time. It's been a full day.

Jerking Off Beforehand

One thing you can try before you have sex for the first time, to extend your performance, is to jerk off before you have sex. I am not guaranteeing that this will work, you may still bust a nut in no time flat, but you can try it.

<u>Make sure that you jerk off at least an hour before you plan on having sex</u>. Don't excuse yourself right before you stick it in and go rub it off in the bathroom. That will cause another problem. The aim of this exercise is to lower your hormone levels to a point where it takes you longer to cum, but not so low that you can't get a hard on.

If you are worried that you will not be able to get hard, well you can rest easy on that fact. You, as a strapping young man should be able to recover and get another hard on in under thirty minutes. It's up to you whether or not to try it. I did, however, it made no difference in the end – I too was a two pump chump.

Nice And Simple

As a young man ready to lose his virginity, you should work towards the aim of having nice and simple sex. Don't get too fancy. Don't try sixteen positions. Don't try out some sexual move that your friend taught you. Just aim for nice, basic, sexual intercourse and a nice quick orgasm. Keep it basic. There will be time for showing off later as your skill, control and familiarity with sex increase.

There Are Two Kinds Of Sex

As you have been reading through this book, you may have noticed that I like to knock your high school health education. This is really true because it is the only place that you are guaranteed to get any education on sex and they don't teach you any of the really practical stuff that you need to know to become a good lover. That is why we have men in this world who think it is OK to listen to a football game while they fuck their wife. True story from a friend. Well, it isn't OK and sex education should be ashamed.

This section is going to teach you another one of those critical facts that you need to know and haven't been taught. That is that there are two kinds of sex and you need to be capable of doing both and switching back and forth.

The first type of sex is what people often refer to as "lovemaking". This type of sex is slow, gentle, tender and passionate. There is lots of kissing and embracing. You are close to your lover. You can feel her skin on your and if things are going slowly you will feel her heartbeat too. This is the kind of sex when people (including this author) whisper things like "I love you" to one another. This type of sex nourishes our souls and bond us together with our lover.

The other kind of sex, for lack of a better term, I am going to call wild sex. Wild sex is animal passion unleashed. This is the kind of sex you have when your partner jumps you and rips your clothes off. This sex happens when you bend your girlfriend over or when there is hair pulling and biting. When you are fucking each other so hard that you fall off the bed, chances are that you are engaged in wild sex. This type of sex is just as important and healthy as love making. In fact, the two exist as opposite and complimentary to each other. While lovemaking nourishes our souls, wild sex satisfies our need to play and let loose. Sometimes we all just need a good fucking and that is where wild sex comes in. It also allows us to assert ourselves or submit to our lovers as our mood and relationships dictate. Make no mistake, both are very healthy and very necessary in a healthy, fun, loving, emotionally satisfying sex life.

However!!! However, wild sex is not what you should be looking for or planning when you are losing your virginity. You should be working to build a healthy, supporting bond with your partner. Losing your virginity is scary and important. You are going to want to feel accepted and embraced. You are also going to want to feel connected to her. Trust me, for her it will be very important to feel connected to you and getting bent over and fucked while she can't even look at her lover will not do that. For both you and her, focus on lovemaking.

As a last note, I should also say that wild sex is only possible when you have built a bond with lovemaking. Once trust has been established and there is a solid foundation to a sexual relationship, then, and only then can you start having the wild, playful sex. Start with lovemaking and the rest will follow young man.

Forget Porn

Porn is ubiquitous in Western culture these days, and if you're reading this book, there is a damn good chance that you've seen a stroke film or two in your day. Thank you very much internet. When I was going through what you are now, we had to buy used magazines that had been pilfered from our friends dad's closets. Oh how the times have changed. Well forget this old fart's pining for the good ol' days. Let's discuss porn and how it fits into losing your virginity.

There is a good chance that you have watched porn, like I said. Since this is really your only experience with actual sex at this point, it would not be unnatural for you to plan to act, while you are losing your viriginty, like the men in the porn scenes you've watched. You might be planning to cum on her tits or pussy. You might be planning to slap your cock (gently of course) on any number of your female companions body parts. Clit, tits, face and ass all come to mine. I know for a fact I have seen that in pornos. You may pull her hair, slap her ass or bend her over. Etc., etc., etc.

Well, don't. I made this mistake. I laugh now about the time I lost my virginity and pulled out to cum all over my girlfriend. I didn't understand the look on her face at the time, but I sure do now.

Girls don't like to get cummed on as a rule, and the sure as hell will not admit to it even if they do. Especially when you are losing your virginity to them. If they ask, fine. Have fun. However, until a girl specifically asks you to cum on her, just don't. Best to cum in that condom you are wearing.

Same goes with slapping your cock anywhere. Slapping their clits can hurt. They really don't like that. It's like hitting you in the balls. Slapping your cock on a girls tits and face really just makes them feel degraded, and as a rule of thumb, girls who feel degraded won't sleep with you again or won't enjoy it if they do. We all want them to enjoy it.

Lastly, spanking and roughhousing can be fun too. However, this is the kind of thing that needs to be discussed with you partner in advance. As a rule, leave this until you have had a good few years of regular vanilla sex under your belt. I'm sure you'll try it. However, you should wait. When you turned sixteen and went to get a license that didn't mean you went to the race track the next day. Same goes with this. Plus, it can really piss a girl off if she is enjoying you fucking her and you suddenly slap her ass out of the blue. That can hurt. Their lovely asses can be sensitive and a pissed off girlfriend with a red handprint on her ass does not go well with your blue balls.

OK, so we've hit a few point about forgetting all of those silly bits that are thrown into porno movies for visual effect. Good. Remember, when you are losing your virginity, you are just going for nice and simple. You can always get complicated later on.

She's Probably Not Going To Cum

Again, I assuming that most of what you know about sex, at this point, comes from porn and your high school health class. This being true, you may be under the impression that your lover is going to start cumming the second that you slip your cock into them. I know this is what I was expecting.

Well, I have some bad news for you there too. This is almost definitely not going to happen and if it does, she's faking. You need to accept a fact that will put you on the course to becoming a wonderful, sought after lover some day. I'm serious.

The fact is this: Most, if not all women, can only cum through stimulation of their clitoris.

It's true. Most women can only cum when their clits are stimulated. They do not cum from vaginal intercourse. The g-spot has never even been proven to exist, medically speaking. Now, maybe there are exceptions to this rule out there. But the truth of the matter is that if you want a girl to cum, you need to stimulate her clit.

Stimulating a woman's clit while you are fucking her is hard to do, and it is almost certainly beyond the ability of a man while he is losing his virginity. You won't be able to focus and while you are fumbling around, there is a greater risk of hurting her clit than there is in stimulating it. For now, and until you are a little more comfortable with sex, hold off on the clitoral stimulation during intercourse.

I am sure that this has raised two questions in your mind. First, you are probably wondering how to go about making your partner cum. You are also probably wondering what women get out of intercourse if they don't orgasm.

The answer to the first question is that you stimulate her clitoris when you aren't fucking her. Usually oral sex is the best for this. However, you can finger her or even bring a vibrator into the bedroom with you. Yes, real men have vibrators for just such a need. Also, some women can orgasm during sex by grinding their clits into their lover's bodies. For this, she should be on top and let her do the work. That way, again, no damage to her clit will occur. If you want to learn more about performing oral sex on a woman, try my other book "The Secret Art Of Eating Pussy: Tips & Tricks To Please Her Every Time", available at all fine book retailers.

As to why women enjoy intercourse, they enjoy it because it feels good. If you don't cum from a blowjob, you can definitely still enjoy it. Women are the same. Sex feels good, they just don't cum. Now, as you become more experienced in the art of love, you should definitely study and learn how to make a woman cum and make sure she does frequently. This is one of those unspoken rules between lovers and what will make you a good lover and a good man. Remember that a Chinese dinner is not over until both of you have eaten your fortune cookies. Orgasms are no different.

Now, I have loaded you up with a lot of info in this section and I am sure I have popped a bit of a fantasy of yours. However, as you are ready to become a man, I think you are comfortable dealing with the truth. In the end, I think it will make you a better lover.

Your Friends Are Full Of Shit

I'm sure that you have guy friends and there is a really good possibility that some of them have already lost their virginity, or claim to have. They may have bragged about their sexual bravado and their conquests. They may have advice for you, the virgin, if they know that you haven't lost your cherry. There may even be pressure on you to hurry up.

Well, I am going to tell you right now that they are probably full of shit. There is a good chance they haven't lost their virginities. That girl from Canada, or in Mexico or the exchange student were all tired, lame stories when I first heard them and they are now too. Even if your friends have lost their virginities, they were probably over pretty quick anyway.

For now, focus on you. Don't worry about where they are, how they lost their virginity or their most likely bullshit stories or advice. Read this book, learn what you need to and when you're ready apply what you've learned. That's it.

Let Her Slip It In

From the diagram in the preceding pages, or from all those blow ups you saw in school, you would think that finding the opening of a woman's pussy is easy. Well, to a beginner, it is a little trickier than that. Yes it can be done, but it's harder to find than you might expect. Pussies, as a general rule, are discreet and those pussy lips keep everything nice and tucked away.

Yes, you can find it. Men have been doing that for a million years. However, in the dark and in your enthusiasm to cross the goal line, you might jam it in prematurely. This won't break her, but it might be a touch uncomfortable for her. Also, if you are too soon and she isn't wet enough, she might chaff a bit.

So, as a gentleman, let her slip it in. Let her decide when the time has come (just wait) and let her guide you into her. She should decide depth and speed. As a result the sex will be much better.

Your Go To First Time Sex Positions

So we have already talked about how you have watched porn. You are probably familiar with every type of sexual position that you can find in the Kama Sutra (If you don't know what that is, look it up online and buy a copy. It's good for later.) You probably know what the reverse cowgirl and the piledriver are. Well, just like porn, you should put all of those positions out of your head.

When you are losing your virginity, there are really only three positions that you should go for. Now, you can try all three of them, and repeat as desired.

Missionary is definitely one of your go to virginity losing positions. First of all, it is intimate. You are face to face at this moment and you feel connected to your partner. This is really nice. You should feel connected to your partner when you lose your virginity. More importantly, there is easy vagina/penis contact. When you are in the missionary position, your cock is right up close to her hoo ha. Ususally all that is needed to slip it in is an adjustment up or down depending on how your pelvises are aligned and how your cock curves.

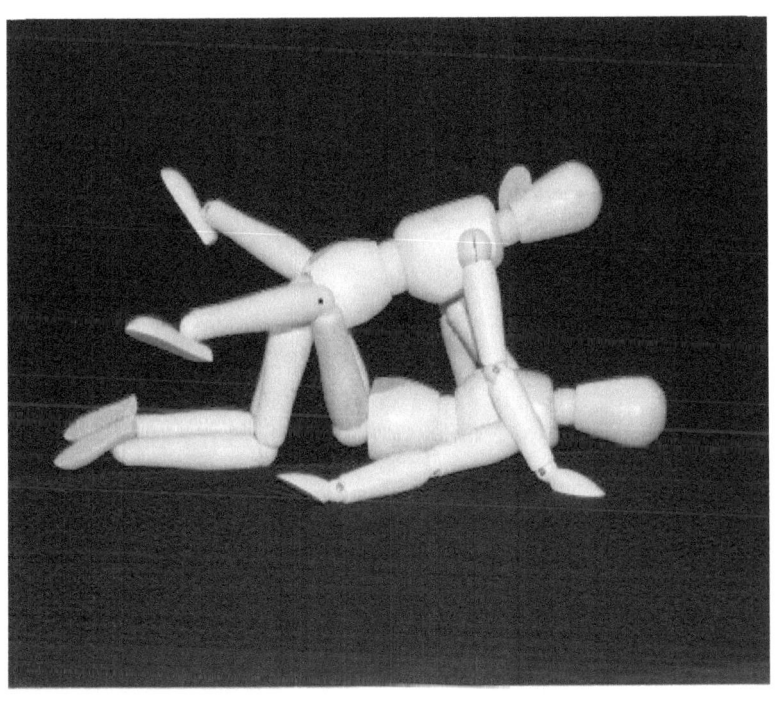

Missionary position is great for easy access to her pussy as well as closeness and face to face to build intimacy.

Cowgirl (not reverse cowgirl) is another position that is great for losing your virginity. Like missionary you are still face to face and very intimate. During the act, you can make out hot and heavy. There is also, still, nice vagina/penis contact. It is really easy to slip it in during cowgirl sex. The advantage of cowgirl sex is that with the woman on top, she is in control of penetration and can regulate how deep and how fast your cock is going into her. This is very important if she is a virgin as well and makes this position the one I would recommend to start with. This also puts her in control and helps her relax as well as making any "losing her virginity pain" as comfortable as possible. If she is a virgin too, you should definitely start here.

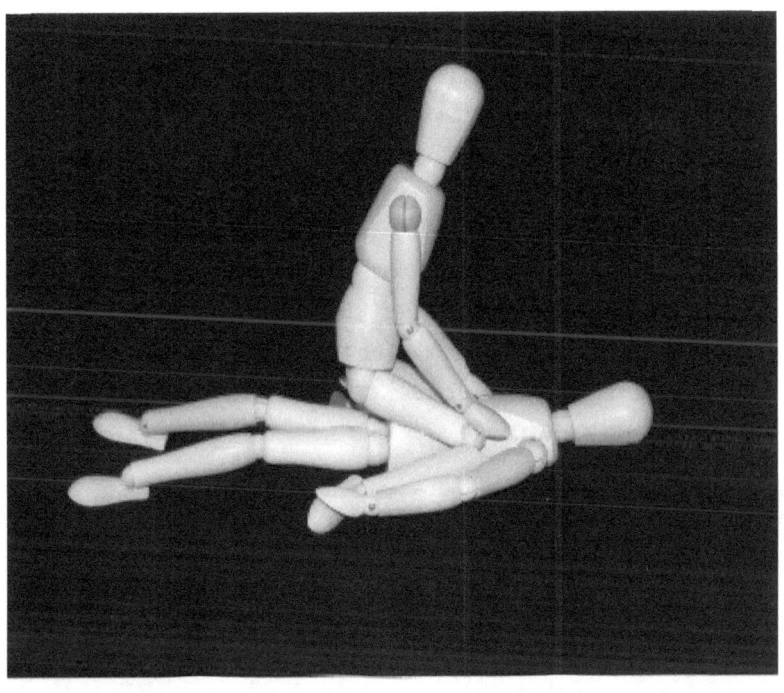

Cowgirl is a great position to lose your virginity. She is in control of how deep penetration is as well as how fast. This position maximizes her comfort but still allows for deep intimacy.

The last position that I would recommend for you is doggystyle. Doggystyle is a lot of fun and more importantly, the position gives you a lot of access to her bikini zone. This can make it a lot easy for you to find her pussy. No more fumbling about like a novice. The one downside to doggystyle is that the intimacy is less than the other two positions that I have mentioned. However, doggystyle can be a lot more vigorous that the other two as well. If your girl is ready to just get fucked, then this is your go to position for sure.

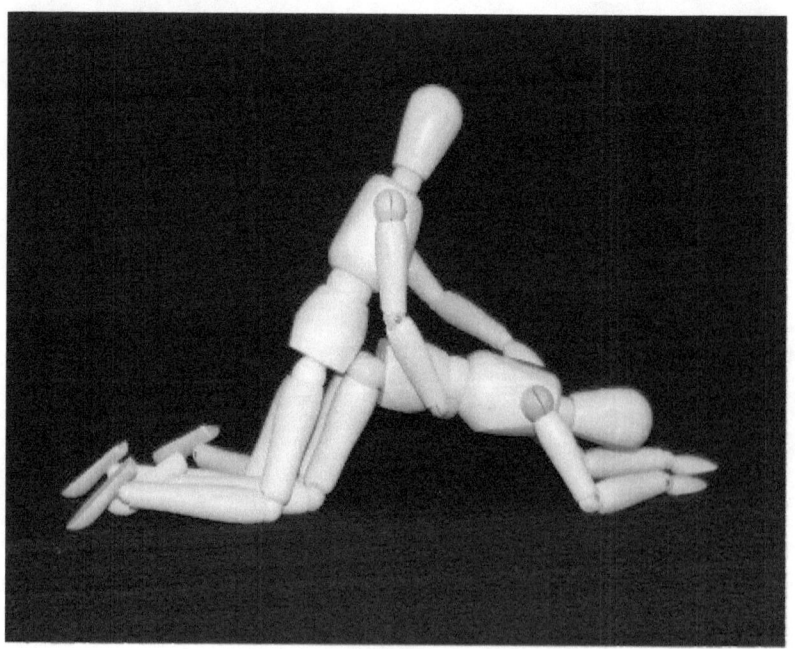

Doggystyle loses out on the intimact. However, the body positioning makes for easy penetration and access to her pussy.

Leave Her Ass Alone

OK. I'm going to burst another one of your bubbles here. Girls don't like to get fucked in the ass. Most of them will try it at one point in their lives, usually at the behest of a nagging boyfriend. However, very, very few of them actually enjoy it or do it after that. Truth be told, it hurts! Also, honestly, it's not fun. I'm going to tell you a story here to illustrate my point.

Let's say I have a friend and this friend and his girlfriend were being "amorous". Well, long story short, they started to have anal sex. He came and then he pulled out. Well, it was at this point that his lady friend had an accident in the bed. Turns out she had been a little backed up and all that anal sex had knocked something lose. Well, now you can see how it can be not fun. Pretty hard to keep your cock hard when your lady friend has just stained your sheets.

So, when you are lucky enough in life to have found a woman who will let you stick it in her pussy, you should just be satisfied with that. Trust me. It will be years before you really get good at just having regular sex with a woman. Focus on that for now.

Possible Bumps In The Road

When a satellite get's launched, there is always the possibility that things will go wrong. Well, I don't want you to get hung up on this, but things can go wrong with sex too. There are three common problems that I want to address with you, like an adult, so you can be aware of them, not panic if they happen and work to correct and overcome them.

Impotence-At some point, in every man's life, he's rearing to go and his cock just isn't. It can be for a lot of reasons. It can be because it needs a break. It can be because he's drunk. I personally have lost my stiffy when I have a lot on my mind and I can't concentrate. It can be psychological, physical, mysterious and frustrating.

The key to overcoming some sort of limp cock situation is to remain calm. If you panic, it's over and everything is lost. Frequently, whatever problem your cock was having will work itself out on its own if you just give it a minute. Try making out with her for a few minutes, or finger or eat her pussy a bit. Don't try and have her blow you. That only puts more pressure on you and will often result in a bad time.

If the worst comes to pass and it's just not happening, tell her you weren't expecting to be making love to her tonight and that you jerked off eight times earlier. Tell her you find her really attractive and that you want to cuddle and try again later. Unfortunately, impotence can hurt a woman's ego as much as a man. Often the look at it as you don't find them attractive. They have no idea how much of an independent mind your cock has. If it just isn't happening, cuddle and bond. You'll get over it, or more than likely, it will start to grow hard on its own.

Dry Pussy-Well, if you haven't followed my advice and had lot and lots and lots of foreplay, you need to go back and get to work. You can't build a house without pouring a foundation. However, it is entirely possible that your lady friend is having her own version of impotence. Maybe she is nervous too. If this is the case, remain calm. If you have followed my instructions and stocked your sex room as I told you, just reach over and grab a bottle of that water based lubricant.

A man who has never applied lube to a pussy will be very tempted to go nuts and pour half the bottle in. No! No! No! A dab will do you. Think like the size of a dime. Apply this amount to the end of your index and middle finger and ever so gently rub it in her pussy. Notice that I said **IN** not **ON** her pussy. You want it in her vagina. If you spread it all on her clit, you're just wasting it. If you need to, refer back to the diagram from before.

Premature Ejaculation-This one can be a bit embarrassing and messy. There is always the chance that you will bust your nut from sheer excitement before you ever get a chance to slip it into your girl. Well, shit happens. If you came all over her, remember you're a gentleman, and get her a towel. A gentleman always gets his girl a towel when she's cleaning up sperm.

First and foremost pretend you're a politician. Stay calm and take control of the message again. Look at your girl and say "Damn. I'm sorry about that but I just got so turned on by you that I couldn't control myself." That line will buy you a lot of time. It turns your embarrassing moment into a compliment that she can brag to her friends about behind your back. Once you've done that, you're back on the horse. Start kissing her, and resume foreplay, maybe even oral sex, until you're ready to go again. Trust me you are young and virile, it won't be long.

Don't get hung up on what can go wrong when we are talking about losing your virginity. The gas tank on you're car can explode or you can get into a car accident. A lot of things **CAN** happen, but most of the time they don't. I'm sure that your first time will go perfectly, if not briefly. However, now that you have read this section, you are well prepared if something unpredictable happens. You'll bounce back and be fucking like a champ in no time!

After You've Lost Your Virginity

95% of the work to lose your virginity is done before you even get your girlfriend naked. However, the 5% you do afterward is very important. That is what makes the difference between you getting to have regular sex with this woman because you are a giving, caring, sensitive lover and having this be a one time thing because you're an asshole. So sit up, pay attention. We're almost done but I've got a last few important things to say.

Cum Again

You are a young man in the prime of life. You should feel pretty good about yourself. You've done it. You've lost your cherry. I'm willing to bet a lot of money that the whole episode took a few minutes at the longest. No worries. Once it's over and you feel your cock start to point north again, feel free to re-wrap with a fresh condom and plunge back into that pussy. Losing your virginity is only the first step in a hopefully, long lifetime of fucking. No use wasting time. Get back in there and feel free to cum again!

Cuddling

When I was young and done with sex, I would hop up, clean up and get on with my day. Honestly, I was a bit of a poor lover. Don't make the same mistake I did. You should stay and cuddle with your girl for as long as she wants.

Women need the intimacy after sex (men do too, they just hate to admit it). This is the time when emotions are high, especially after orgasm, and when we can feel as close to one another as is possible. Take a pause and don't rush up. Don't rush to shower and wash all of her juices off of you either, this can be insulting. Instead, bask in the afterglow and enjoy. If you have to lie in a wet spot, shut up and do it. If you simply pledge to let her get up, out of the bed first, you'll be fine and much more sexually sophisticated than just about any man your age. Try and earn the reputation of "Cuddle Bug".

Get Off Your Ass And Get Her A Towel

Sex can be a bit on the sloppy side as you will soon learn. There are a lot of bodily fluids involved. Don't get me wrong, the messier the sex, usually the better it was. Anyway, when it is all over, there are some clean up issues. You need to slip off your condom and dispose of it and she will most likely want to wipe up her pussy. No problems there, except the towels are in the bathroom. Well, after cuddling for a few minutes, get up like a gentleman and get her a towel. This lovely woman, whoever she is, just let you fuck her. The least you can do is get up and get that towel for her. When she has wiped up a bit, get right back to cuddling.

You are a young man in the prime of life. You should feel pretty good about yourself. You've done it. You've lost your cherry. I'm willing to bet a lot of money that the whole episode took a few minutes at the longest. No worries. Once it's over and you feel your cock start to point north again, feel free to re-wrap with a fresh condom and plunge back into that pussy. Losing your virginity is only the first step in a hopefully, long lifetime of fucking. No use wasting time. Get back in there and feel free to cum again!

Cuddling

When I was young and done with sex, I would hop up, clean up and get on with my day. Honestly, I was a bit of a poor lover. Don't make the same mistake I did. You should stay and cuddle with your girl for as long as she wants.

Women need the intimacy after sex (men do too, they just hate to admit it). This is the time when emotions are high, especially after orgasm, and when we can feel as close to one another as is possible. Take a pause and don't rush up. Don't rush to shower and wash all of her juices off of you either, this can be insulting. Instead, bask in the afterglow and enjoy. If you have to lie in a wet spot, shut up and do it. If you simply pledge to let her get up, out of the bed first, you'll be fine and much more sexually sophisticated than just about any man your age. Try and earn the reputation of "Cuddle Bug".

Get Off Your Ass And Get Her A Towel

Sex can be a bit on the sloppy side as you will soon learn. There are a lot of bodily fluids involved. Don't get me wrong, the messier the sex, usually the better it was. Anyway, when it is all over, there are some clean up issues. You need to slip off your condom and dispose of it and she will most likely want to wipe up her pussy. No problems there, except the towels are in the bathroom. Well, after cuddling for a few minutes, get up like a gentleman and get her a towel. This lovely woman, whoever she is, just let you fuck her. The least you can do is get up and get that towel for her. When she has wiped up a bit, get right back to cuddling.

A Gentleman Is Discreet

Once the big moment is over, you may be tempted to go and brag to all your friends. You might call, text or post on any number of social media sites. Stop!!! Don't do this. Remember what I said about women being sensitive about the number of partners they've had and their sexualities as a whole. If you go and brag to all your buddies, there is a good chance that someone, somewhere will make her feel like a slut. This will make her legs snap shut like a bear trap.

You are left with a choice. Do you want to be the guy who got laid once and all his friends know it? Or, do you want to be the guy who bends his girlfriend over the kitchen table while his parents are away every Tuesday and Thursday? The choice is yours and yours alone, but a gentleman is discreet.

The Journey Has Only Just Begun

In all honesty, your first sexual experience is like any prototype. It's crude, not quite 100% right but shows lots of potential. It wasn't perfect, in fact it was far from it. You took your first step, but there are many more to come.

At this point, your sex education has only just begun. There is much more to do. This is the time that you need to be hitting the books. You lost your virginity, but now you need to learn about pussy eating, female orgasm, group sex, BDSM, etc., etc.

You're like Columbus the day after he discovered America. You've done a lot, but a whole world lies at your feet for exploration. Hit up your local bookstore or even library and get to work. Never forget that good lovers are just bad lovers who studied really hard. Which one do you want to be?

-C.W. Pollard

www.ingramcontent.com/pod-product-compliance
Lightning Source LLC
Chambersburg PA
CBHW021239280526
45784CB00005B/2153